Metabolism Plan Beginners Guide Made Easy

Lifestyle Factors Affecting Metabolism

By

Fredo Alvin

Copyright@2023

Table of Contents

CHAPTER 1

Introduction to Metabolism

1.1 What is Metabolism?

Metabolism is a complex and fundamental process that occurs in every living organism, from plants and animals to humans. It is the set of chemical reactions that take place within cells to sustain life and maintain the body's functions. Metabolism is the cornerstone of life, enabling organisms to extract energy from the environment and use it to carry out essential processes such as growth, repair, reproduction, and movement.

At its core, metabolism is all about the transformation of matter and energy. It involves breaking down large molecules, such as carbohydrates, fats, and proteins, into smaller components, releasing energy in the process. This energy is then harnessed to fuel cellular activities and the overall functioning of the body. Additionally, metabolism involves building complex molecules from smaller units, a process known as anabolism, which requires energy input.

Metabolism is a dynamic and tightly regulated process that adapts to the body's needs, environmental changes, and available resources. Several factors influence an individual's metabolism, including age, sex, genetics, body composition, physical activity, diet, hormonal balance, and overall health status. For instance, someone with a higher percentage of lean muscle mass tends to have a higher basal metabolic rate (BMR) because muscle cells require more energy to maintain than fat cells.

The primary purpose of metabolism is to maintain homeostasis, the stable internal environment necessary for the body's survival and proper functioning. This equilibrium ensures that cells receive the necessary nutrients and energy while removing waste products and harmful substances.

The main components involved in metabolism are enzymes, which act as biological catalysts to speed up chemical reactions without being consumed in the process. Enzymes are specific to particular reactions and help regulate the metabolic pathways, ensuring that the right reactions occur at the right time and in the right amounts.

Metabolism can be divided into two major categories: catabolism and anabolism.

1.1.1 Catabolism

Catabolism involves the breakdown of larger molecules into smaller ones, resulting in the release of energy. The primary purpose of catabolic reactions is to obtain energy and building blocks for anabolic processes. For example, during the digestion of food, complex carbohydrates are broken down into simple sugars, fats into fatty acids, and proteins into amino acids, all of which can be further utilized to produce energy or synthesize new molecules.

The energy released during catabolic processes is often stored in the form of adenosine triphosphate (ATP), a molecule that acts as the primary energy currency in cells. ATP is used to power various cellular activities, such as muscle contraction, nerve impulse transmission, and biosynthesis.

1.1.2 Anabolism

Anabolism involves the synthesis of larger molecules from smaller ones, requiring energy input. This process is essential for growth, tissue repair, and the production of complex molecules like proteins, nucleic acids, and cellular structures. Anabolic reactions typically utilize the energy stored in ATP to drive the construction of new molecules and facilitate cellular growth and repair.

The balance between catabolism and anabolism is critical for overall health and well-being. When the rate of catabolism exceeds anabolism, the body may break down more tissue than it can rebuild, leading to muscle wasting and other health issues. On the other hand, if anabolism predominates, excess energy may be stored as fat, potentially leading to weight gain and related health problems.

metabolism is a dynamic and intricate process that governs how our bodies obtain, utilize, and store energy for various cellular activities. Understanding metabolism is crucial for maintaining a healthy lifestyle, managing weight, and preventing metabolic disorders. By nourishing our bodies with appropriate nutrition, engaging in regular physical activity, and adopting healthy lifestyle habits, we can optimize our metabolism and promote overall well-being.

1.2 Importance of Understanding Your Metabolism

Understanding your metabolism is of utmost importance as it plays a central role in your overall health, well-being, and body composition. Here are several key reasons why gaining insight into your metabolism is crucial:

1. Weight Management: One of the primary reasons people seek to understand their metabolism is its significant impact on weight management. Metabolism determines how

many calories your body burns at rest (basal metabolic rate) and during physical activities. If you have a slower metabolism, you may burn fewer calories, making it easier to gain weight or harder to lose weight. By contrast, having a faster metabolism might allow you to burn more calories, aiding in weight loss efforts. Understanding your metabolic rate can help you tailor your diet and exercise plans to achieve and maintain a healthy weight.

2. Personalized Nutrition: Different individuals have unique nutritional needs based on their metabolic rates and overall energy requirements. Knowing your metabolism can

help you personalize your diet by determining the ideal balance of macronutrients (proteins, carbohydrates, and fats) and portion sizes. It can also guide you in making informed choices about the frequency and timing of meals to keep your energy levels stable and support your overall health.

3. Fitness and Exercise: Understanding your metabolism can influence your exercise choices and fitness goals. People with higher metabolic rates might find it easier to build muscle and improve athletic performance. On the other hand, individuals with slower metabolisms might benefit from certain types of

exercises, such as high-intensity interval training (HIIT), which can boost metabolism and burn more calories in a shorter amount of time.

4. Energy Levels and Fatigue: Metabolism determines how efficiently your body converts food into energy. If your metabolism is sluggish, you may experience low energy levels and persistent fatigue. By understanding your metabolism, you can identify potential issues and adopt lifestyle changes to optimize your energy levels and combat fatigue.

5. Preventing Metabolic Disorders: A proper understanding of metabolism

can also help identify potential risk factors for metabolic disorders, such as diabetes, obesity, and cardiovascular diseases. With this knowledge, you can take proactive measures to reduce these risks through lifestyle changes, including diet modifications, regular exercise, and stress management.

6. Aging and Hormonal Changes: As we age, our metabolism naturally slows down, which can lead to changes in body composition and energy expenditure. Understanding this process can help you adapt your lifestyle to accommodate these changes and maintain a healthy weight and body function as you get older.

7. Personal Empowerment:
    Knowledge of your metabolism
    empowers you to take control
    of your health and make
    informed decisions about your
    diet, exercise, and lifestyle
    choices. Rather than relying on
    generic advice, understanding
    your individual metabolic
    profile allows you to create a
    personalized plan that suits
    your unique needs and goals.

understanding your metabolism is
essential for managing weight,
optimizing nutrition and fitness,
maintaining energy levels, and
preventing metabolic disorders. By
gaining insights into how your body
processes energy and nutrients, you
can make informed decisions about
your lifestyle, leading to improved
overall health and well-being. It is

important to consult with healthcare professionals or registered dietitians to obtain accurate assessments and guidance for understanding and optimizing your metabolism.

CHAPTER 2

The Basics of Metabolism

2.1 Understanding Calories and Energy Balance

Calories and energy balance are fundamental concepts when it comes to understanding metabolism and how our bodies regulate weight. Here's a breakdown of these concepts:

2.1.1 Calories

A calorie is a unit of measurement for energy. In the context of nutrition, it refers to the amount of energy obtained from food and beverages when our bodies break them down during digestion. The energy stored in food is used by the body to perform various functions, such as maintaining body temperature, supporting organ function, physical activity, and cellular processes.

The three primary macronutrients in our diet contribute calories:

- Carbohydrates: 1 gram = 4 calories

- Proteins: 1 gram = 4 calories

- Fats: 1 gram = 9 calories

When we consume more calories than our bodies need to perform daily activities and maintain basic functions, the excess energy is stored in the form of fat. On the other hand, if we consume fewer calories than our bodies require, the stored fat is used as a source of energy, leading to weight loss.

2.1.2 Energy Balance

Energy balance refers to the relationship between the number of calories consumed through food and beverages (energy intake) and the number of calories expended by the body (energy expenditure). When energy intake equals energy expenditure, the body is in a state of energy balance, and weight remains stable.

There are three possible states of energy balance:

- Positive Energy Balance: When energy intake exceeds energy expenditure, the body is in a positive energy balance. This leads to weight gain as excess calories are stored as fat.

- Negative Energy Balance:
  When energy expenditure
  exceeds energy intake, the body
  is in a negative energy balance.
  This results in weight loss as
  the body taps into its fat stores
  for additional energy.

- Neutral Energy Balance: When
  energy intake matches energy
  expenditure, the body is in a
  neutral energy balance, and
  weight remains stable.

2.1.3 Factors Affecting Energy Balance

Several factors influence energy balance and, consequently, weight management. These factors include:

- Basal Metabolic Rate (BMR):
  BMR is the number of calories
  the body needs to maintain
  basic physiological functions

while at rest, such as breathing, circulating blood, and maintaining body temperature. BMR accounts for the majority of energy expenditure in most individuals.

- Physical Activity: The number of calories expended through physical activity varies depending on the type, duration, and intensity of the exercise. Regular physical activity increases energy expenditure and can help with weight management.

- Thermic Effect of Food (TEF): TEF refers to the energy expended during the digestion, absorption, and processing of nutrients in the body. The body uses energy to break down food into its usable components, and different macronutrients have varying thermic effects.

- Non-Exercise Activity Thermogenesis (NEAT): NEAT encompasses the energy expended during everyday activities that are not considered formal exercise, such as fidgeting, walking, and household chores.

- Hormonal Factors: Hormones play a role in regulating appetite, hunger, and satiety, influencing energy intake. Hormonal imbalances can affect energy balance and weight regulation.

2.2 Metabolic Rate and Its Factors

Metabolic rate refers to the rate at which the body uses energy (burns calories) to sustain its various functions and processes. It can be broken down into several components:

2.2.1 Basal Metabolic Rate (BMR)

Basal Metabolic Rate (BMR) is the energy expenditure required to maintain essential physiological functions while the body is at rest. These functions include breathing, circulating blood, maintaining body temperature, and supporting organ function. BMR accounts for the largest portion of an individual's total energy expenditure, usually representing around 60-75% of the total.

Several factors influence BMR:

- Age: BMR tends to decrease with age as lean muscle mass typically decreases while body fat increases.

- Body Composition: Individuals with higher muscle mass generally have a higher BMR because muscle tissue requires more energy to maintain than fat tissue.

- Sex: In general, men tend to have a higher BMR than women, mainly due to differences in body composition and hormone levels.

- Genetics: Genetic factors can play a role in determining an individual's BMR.

2.2.2 Resting Metabolic Rate (RMR)

Resting Metabolic Rate (RMR) is similar to BMR but is measured under less strict conditions. While BMR is typically measured under controlled laboratory conditions, RMR is measured under more relaxed circumstances, such as waking up in the morning but before engaging in any physical activity. RMR accounts for a slightly higher percentage of total energy expenditure compared to BMR.

2.2.3 Total Daily Energy Expenditure (TDEE)

Total Daily Energy Expenditure (TDEE) represents the total number of calories an individual burns in a day, taking into account all activities, including physical activity and the thermic effect of food. TDEE is the sum of BMR/RMR, physical activity energy expenditure, thermic effect of food, and NEAT.

Factors affecting Total Daily Energy Expenditure include:

- Physical Activity Level: More physically active individuals will have a higher TDEE.

- Thermic Effect of Food: The process of digesting, absorbing, and processing nutrients from food contributes to TDEE.

- Non-Exercise Activity Thermogenesis (NEAT): Everyday activities like walking, standing, and fidgeting can contribute significantly to TDEE.

It's important to note that individual metabolic rates can vary significantly due to factors like age, sex, genetics, body composition, and lifestyle. Understanding these factors can help individuals make informed decisions about their dietary choices, exercise routines, and weight management goals. Additionally, any significant changes in lifestyle, such as starting a new exercise program or adjusting one's diet, may impact metabolic rate and energy balance. Therefore, it is essential to approach any changes with a balanced and sustainable approach to maintain overall health and well-being.

2.3 Different Types of Metabolism

When referring to "different types of metabolism," it usually pertains to the variations in how individuals' bodies process and utilize energy. Several factors can influence an individual's metabolic rate and how their body manages energy. Here are some key considerations regarding different types of metabolism:

1. Fast Metabolism: People with a fast metabolism are often able to burn calories at a higher rate than average, leading to a quicker energy expenditure.

Several factors may contribute to a fast metabolism, including:

- Genetics: Some individuals are genetically predisposed to have a higher basal metabolic rate (BMR) or efficient energy expenditure.

- Lean Muscle Mass: Having more lean muscle mass increases the body's metabolic needs because muscle tissue requires more energy to maintain than fat tissue.

- Physical Activity: Regular exercise and physical activity can boost metabolic rate, especially when it includes strength training and high-intensity exercises.

- Age: Younger individuals tend to have faster metabolisms, but this rate naturally declines with age.

2. Slow Metabolism: Conversely, people with a slow metabolism may burn calories at a slower rate, leading to potentially easier weight gain or difficulty losing weight. Factors contributing to a slow metabolism may include:

- Genetics: Genetics can play a role in determining an individual's metabolic rate and how efficiently their body uses energy.

- Low Muscle Mass: A lower amount of lean muscle mass can result in a slower metabolism as there is less tissue requiring energy.

- Sedentary Lifestyle: A lack of physical activity and exercise can lead to a decrease in metabolic rate over time.

- Age: As individuals age, their metabolism tends to slow down, which can contribute to weight gain if dietary habits remain unchanged.

3. Adaptive Metabolism: Some individuals may experience what is known as adaptive metabolism. This occurs when the body adapts to changes in calorie intake or physical activity levels. For example, during periods of calorie restriction or dieting, the body may adjust its metabolic rate to conserve energy, making weight loss more challenging. This adaptive response is

thought to be an evolutionary mechanism to protect against starvation.

4. Endomorph, Mesomorph, and Ectomorph Body Types: In some discussions, people's body types are categorized into endomorph, mesomorph, and ectomorph. These classifications suggest that different body types may have different metabolic tendencies:

- Endomorph: Endomorphs are often described as having a higher tendency to store body fat and may have a slower metabolism. They typically have a rounder physique with a greater proportion of body fat.

- Mesomorph: Mesomorphs tend to have a more muscular and

athletic build. They may have a faster metabolism and find it easier to build and maintain muscle mass.

- Ectomorph: Ectomorphs are usually characterized by a lean and slender body type. They often have a faster metabolism and may find it challenging to gain weight or muscle.

It's important to note that these body type classifications are generalized and may not fully capture the complexity of an individual's metabolism. Moreover, multiple factors influence metabolism, and individuals may have characteristics from more than one body type.

In reality, metabolism is highly individual and influenced by a combination of genetic,

environmental, lifestyle, and
hormonal factors. While some people
may naturally have a faster or slower
metabolism, lifestyle choices, such as
regular exercise and a balanced diet,
can play a crucial role in optimizing
metabolism and maintaining overall
health. Additionally, metabolism can
change over time due to various
factors, making it essential to adopt
sustainable and healthy habits for
long-term well-being.

CHAPTER 3

Assessing Your Metabolic Health

3.1 Identifying Signs of a Fast or Slow Metabolism

Identifying signs of a fast or slow metabolism can provide insights into how efficiently your body processes and utilizes energy. However, it's essential to remember that metabolism is a complex process influenced by various factors, and these signs are general indicators rather than definitive assessments. Here are some signs that may suggest whether you have a relatively fast or slow metabolism:

Signs of a Fast Metabolism:

1. Weight Management: If you find it challenging to gain weight or have difficulty maintaining body fat, it could be a sign of a faster metabolism. Individuals with fast metabolisms often burn calories quickly, leading to a leaner body composition.

2. Constant Hunger: A fast metabolism can result in increased appetite and frequent hunger. Your body may require more energy to maintain its functions and activities, leading to the need for more frequent meals and snacks.

3. High Energy Levels: People with fast metabolisms often experience higher energy levels

throughout the day. They may feel more energized and alert, even without consuming large meals.

4. Tolerance for Carbohydrates: Individuals with fast metabolisms may tolerate carbohydrates well, as their bodies efficiently process and utilize glucose for energy.

5. Quick Digestion: If you have a fast metabolism, you may notice that your body processes and digests food relatively quickly, resulting in more frequent bowel movements.

Signs of a Slow Metabolism:

1. Weight Management: Difficulty losing weight or a tendency to gain weight easily may indicate a slower

metabolism. With a slower metabolic rate, your body might store more calories as fat.

2. Fatigue and Low Energy Levels: Slower metabolism can lead to reduced energy levels and feelings of fatigue, as the body expends energy at a slower rate.

3. Slower Digestion: If you have a slow metabolism, you may experience slower digestion, leading to feelings of fullness and bloating after meals.

4. Cold Sensitivity: Slower metabolism can affect how efficiently your body regulates body temperature, making you feel colder more easily.

5. Difficulty Tolerating Carbohydrates: Individuals

with slower metabolisms may experience fluctuations in blood sugar levels and find it more challenging to process carbohydrates efficiently.

It's important to recognize that these signs are not definitive indicators of metabolic rate and should not be used as a sole basis for assessing metabolic health. Many factors influence metabolism, and individual variations are significant. If you have concerns about your metabolic health or weight management, it's advisable to consult with a healthcare professional, registered dietitian, or certified nutritionist for a comprehensive assessment.

3.2 Tools for Measuring Metabolic Rate

Various tools and methods can help assess metabolic rate. While some approaches provide accurate and direct measurements, others offer estimates based on formulas and data inputs. Here are some common tools used for measuring metabolic rate:

1. Indirect Calorimetry: Indirect calorimetry is a precise method for measuring metabolic rate. It involves measuring the body's oxygen consumption and carbon dioxide production during rest or physical activity. From these measurements, the number of calories burned can be calculated. Indirect calorimetry is often performed in specialized laboratories and medical settings.

2. Basal Metabolic Rate (BMR)
    Calculators: BMR calculators
    estimate the number of calories
    your body burns at rest based
    on factors such as age, sex,
    weight, height, and activity
    level. While these calculators
    are convenient and easy to use,
    they provide estimates rather
    than direct measurements.

3. Metabolic Analyzers: Portable
    metabolic analyzers use
    technology similar to indirect
    calorimetry to estimate resting
    metabolic rate (RMR). These
    devices can be used in various
    settings, including fitness
    centers and sports performance
    facilities.

4. Activity Trackers: Some
    advanced activity trackers and
    fitness wearables claim to

estimate total daily energy expenditure (TDEE) based on various inputs, including heart rate, movement, and personal data. While these estimates can be helpful for tracking trends, they may not be as accurate as direct measurements.

5. Medical Devices: In certain medical conditions, doctors may use specialized medical devices, such as respiratory gas analyzers, to measure metabolic rate for diagnostic purposes.

When using tools to assess metabolic rate, it's essential to consider the limitations and potential inaccuracies associated with each method. For the most accurate assessment and personalized guidance, consulting with a healthcare professional or registered dietitian is recommended.

They can help interpret the results, consider individual factors, and provide tailored recommendations to optimize metabolic health and overall well-being.

3.3 Interpreting Results and What They Mean

Interpreting metabolic rate results is essential for understanding your body's energy needs and overall metabolic health. The interpretation will depend on the method used to measure metabolic rate and the specific context of your health and lifestyle goals. Here's a guide on interpreting metabolic rate results and what they may mean:

1. Indirect Calorimetry Results: If you underwent indirect

calorimetry, which provides direct measurements of oxygen consumption and carbon dioxide production, the results will give an accurate estimation of your resting metabolic rate (RMR) or basal metabolic rate (BMR). The RMR/BMR represents the number of calories your body burns at rest to maintain essential physiological functions.

Interpreting Indirect Calorimetry Results:

- Low RMR/BMR: A lower-than-average RMR/BMR might indicate a slower metabolism, meaning your body requires fewer calories at rest. This could make it easier to gain weight or harder to lose weight, and you may need to adjust your calorie intake and physical activity to reach your weight management goals.

- High RMR/BMR: A higher-than-average RMR/BMR suggests a faster metabolism, indicating that your body burns more calories at rest. This may make it easier to maintain or lose weight, but you still need to maintain a balanced diet and exercise routine for overall health.

2. Basal Metabolic Rate (BMR) Calculators: If you used online BMR calculators, the results provide an estimated resting metabolic rate based on your age, sex, weight, height, and activity level. Remember that these are estimates and not direct measurements.

Interpreting BMR Calculator Results:

- Low Estimated BMR: A lower estimated BMR might suggest a slower metabolism, but it's important to remember that these calculators provide estimates and may not accurately represent your actual metabolic rate. If you struggle with weight management or experience persistent fatigue, it's best to consult a healthcare professional for a comprehensive assessment.

- High Estimated BMR: A higher estimated BMR suggests a faster metabolism, but, again, it's important to consider these results as estimates. Your actual metabolic rate can be influenced by various factors.

3. Consideration of Individual Factors: It's crucial to interpret metabolic rate results while considering individual factors that influence metabolism, such as:

- Age: Metabolism tends to slow down with age due to muscle loss and hormonal changes.

- Genetics: Genetic factors can impact your natural metabolic rate and how your body processes energy.

- Body Composition: The proportion of muscle mass to fat mass can affect metabolic rate.

- Physical Activity: Regular exercise can boost metabolic rate and contribute to overall energy expenditure.

- Hormonal Imbalances: Hormonal disorders, such as thyroid issues, can influence metabolism.

- Dietary Habits: What and how you eat can affect energy intake and expenditure.

4. Implications for Health and Weight Management: Interpreting metabolic rate results can provide insights into potential weight management challenges or how your body responds to different dietary and exercise approaches. However, it's essential to approach this information with a holistic view of overall health and well-being.

For personalized guidance and recommendations based on your

metabolic rate results and health goals, consider consulting with a registered dietitian or healthcare professional. They can help you create a tailored plan that considers your individual needs, preferences, and lifestyle to optimize your metabolic health and achieve your desired health outcomes. Remember that sustainable changes to diet and exercise habits, along with overall healthy lifestyle choices, play key roles in supporting metabolic health and overall well-being.

CHAPTER 4

Fueling Your Metabolism with Nutrition

4.1 The Role of Macros (Proteins, Carbohydrates, Fats)

Macronutrients, also known as macros, are the three main components of our diet that provide energy in the form of calories. They play a crucial role in fueling our metabolism and supporting various physiological functions. Understanding the role of each macronutrient is essential for optimizing metabolic health. Here's a breakdown of the role of proteins, carbohydrates, and fats in metabolism:

1. Proteins: Proteins are composed of amino acids, which are essential for building and repairing tissues, including muscles, organs, and enzymes. The role of proteins in metabolism includes:

- Metabolism Boost: The thermic effect of food (TEF) is the energy required to digest, absorb, and process nutrients. Protein has the highest TEF among all macros, meaning that it requires more energy to be metabolized, effectively boosting your metabolism.

- Muscle Maintenance and Growth: Proteins are crucial for

maintaining and building lean muscle mass. More muscle mass increases the body's basal metabolic rate (BMR) since muscles require energy to be maintained.

- Satiety and Appetite Control: Protein-rich foods tend to promote feelings of fullness and satiety, which can help regulate appetite and reduce overall calorie intake.

Sources of protein include lean meats, poultry, fish, eggs, dairy products, legumes, nuts, and seeds.

2. Carbohydrates: Carbohydrates are the body's primary source of energy. They are broken down into glucose (blood sugar), which provides fuel for the brain, muscles, and other

organs. The role of carbohydrates in metabolism includes:

- Immediate Energy: Carbohydrates are quickly converted into glucose, providing immediate energy for daily activities and exercise.

- Glycogen Storage: Excess glucose is stored as glycogen in the muscles and liver for later use when energy demands are higher.

- Spares Proteins: Adequate carbohydrate intake spares proteins from being used for energy, allowing them to fulfill their essential functions.

Sources of carbohydrates include fruits, vegetables, whole grains, legumes, and starchy foods like potatoes and rice.

3. Fats: Fats are an essential part of a healthy diet, providing a concentrated source of energy and serving as building blocks for cell membranes and hormones. The role of fats in metabolism includes:

- Energy Storage: Fats are the body's most concentrated energy source and provide a long-term energy reserve.

- Absorption of Fat-Soluble Vitamins: Vitamins A, D, E, and K are fat-soluble, meaning they require dietary fats for proper absorption.

- Hormone Production: Fats are precursors to many hormones

involved in metabolism and other physiological processes.

Sources of fats include avocados, nuts, seeds, olive oil, fatty fish, and healthy oils like coconut and flaxseed oil.

Achieving a balanced intake of proteins, carbohydrates, and fats is essential for supporting metabolic health and overall well-being. It's important to remember that individual needs for each macronutrient may vary based on factors such as age, sex, activity level, and health status. Working with a registered dietitian can help you determine the appropriate macronutrient distribution that aligns with your specific goals and health needs.

4.2 The Impact of Micronutrients on Metabolism

In addition to macronutrients, micronutrients are essential vitamins and minerals that play a critical role in supporting metabolism and overall health. These micronutrients act as coenzymes, helping enzymes perform their functions in various metabolic pathways. Here are some key micronutrients and their impact on metabolism:

1. Vitamin B Complex: B vitamins, such as B1 (thiamine), B2 (riboflavin), B3 (niacin), B5 (pantothenic acid), B6 (pyridoxine), B7 (biotin), B9 (folate), and B12 (cobalamin), are vital for energy production and

metabolism. They help convert macronutrients into usable energy, making them essential for the proper functioning of various metabolic pathways.

2. Vitamin C: Vitamin C is an antioxidant that supports immune function and helps the body absorb iron from plant-based sources. It also plays a role in collagen synthesis, which is essential for maintaining healthy skin, bones, and connective tissues.

3. Vitamin D: Vitamin D plays a crucial role in calcium absorption and bone health. It also affects insulin sensitivity and may play a role in metabolic regulation.

4. Calcium: Calcium is essential for muscle function, nerve transmission, and bone health. It also plays a role in various enzymatic reactions involved in metabolism.

5. Magnesium: Magnesium is a cofactor for many enzymes involved in energy production and glucose metabolism. It also supports muscle and nerve function.

6. Zinc: Zinc is involved in numerous metabolic processes, including protein synthesis, immune function, and wound healing.

7. Iron: Iron is a key component of hemoglobin in red blood cells, enabling oxygen transport and energy production. Iron is

vital for maintaining energy levels and preventing anemia.

8. Chromium: Chromium is involved in carbohydrate and lipid metabolism, particularly in enhancing insulin sensitivity.

9. Iodine: Iodine is essential for the production of thyroid hormones, which regulate metabolism and energy expenditure.

A well-balanced and varied diet that includes a wide range of nutrient-dense foods can help ensure adequate intake of these essential micronutrients. Eating a variety of fruits, vegetables, whole grains, lean proteins, and healthy fats can contribute to supporting metabolic health and overall nutrition.

It's important to remember that while macronutrients and micronutrients play critical roles in metabolism, no single nutrient can work in isolation. A balanced and varied diet, combined with regular physical activity and overall healthy lifestyle habits, is essential for optimal metabolic health and well-being. If you have specific health concerns or dietary questions, consider consulting with a registered dietitian or healthcare professional for personalized guidance and recommendations.

4.3 Meal Planning for Optimal Metabolic Function

Meal planning plays a crucial role in supporting optimal metabolic function. Designing balanced and nutritious meals can help regulate blood sugar levels, control appetite, and provide the energy needed for daily activities. Here are some tips for meal planning to promote a healthy metabolism:

1. Balance Macronutrients: Include a combination of proteins, carbohydrates, and fats in each meal. Balancing macronutrients helps stabilize blood sugar levels and provides sustained energy throughout the day. Aim to include lean proteins, whole grains, healthy fats, and a variety of fruits and vegetables in your meals.

2. Prioritize Protein: Ensure each meal contains a good source of protein. Protein-rich foods promote satiety, help maintain lean muscle mass, and have a

higher thermic effect, contributing to a slightly higher metabolic rate.

3. Choose Complex Carbohydrates: opt for complex carbohydrates, such as whole grains, legumes, and vegetables, over refined and sugary options. Complex carbs release energy more gradually, preventing blood sugar spikes and crashes.

4. Incorporate Healthy Fats: Include sources of healthy fats, such as avocados, nuts, seeds, and olive oil. Fats are essential for hormone production and help keep you feeling full and satisfied after meals.

5. Eat Regularly: Avoid long periods of fasting between

meals. Eating regular, balanced meals and snacks throughout the day supports a steady energy supply and prevents extreme hunger, which can lead to overeating.

6. Avoid Highly Processed Foods: Minimize consumption of highly processed foods, sugary beverages, and excessive added sugars. These can lead to blood sugar fluctuations and contribute to metabolic disturbances.

7. Stay Hydrated: Drink an adequate amount of water throughout the day. Staying hydrated support's metabolic function and overall health.

8. Mindful Eating: Practice mindful eating by paying

attention to hunger and fullness cues. Avoid distractions while eating, and take time to savor your meals, promoting better digestion and satisfaction.

9. Plan Ahead: Plan your meals and snacks ahead of time. This can help you make healthier choices and avoid impulsive, less nutritious options when hunger strikes.

10. Control Portion Sizes: Be mindful of portion sizes to prevent overeating. Use smaller plates and listen to your body's hunger and fullness signals to avoid excessive calorie intake.

11. Consider Nutrient Timing: While nutrient timing isn't a strict requirement, some individuals find that spreading

out protein intake throughout the day or consuming carbohydrates around exercise can be beneficial for their metabolism and fitness goals.

12. Individualize Your Plan: Remember that meal planning should be personalized based on your individual needs, preferences, and health goals. Consider consulting with a registered dietitian to create a meal plan that aligns with your specific metabolic needs and lifestyle.

By following this meal planning tips and adopting a balanced and nutritious diet, you can support optimal metabolic function, maintain energy levels, and promote overall well-being. Additionally, coupling a healthy diet with regular physical activity and a well-rounded lifestyle can further enhance your metabolic health and lead to positive long-term results.

CHAPTER 5

Metabolism-Boosting Exercises

5.1 Understanding the Connection Between Exercise and Metabolism

The connection between exercise and metabolism is significant and plays a crucial role in overall health and weight management. Exercise has the potential to boost metabolism in several ways, influencing how the body uses and burns calories. Understanding this connection can help individuals tailor their exercise routines to optimize their metabolic function. Here are some key points to consider:

1. Increased Energy Expenditure: When you engage in physical activity, your body requires additional energy to perform the exercise. This increased energy expenditure can contribute to a higher total daily energy expenditure (TDEE), which includes both basal metabolic rate (BMR) and physical activity energy expenditure.

2. Muscle Mass and Metabolism: Building and maintaining muscle mass is metabolically beneficial. Muscles require more energy to maintain than fat tissue, meaning that individuals with higher muscle mass tend to have higher

BMRs, even at rest. Engaging in resistance training and strength-building exercises can help increase muscle mass and support metabolic health.

3. Post-Exercise Calorie Burn: After a workout, the body may continue to burn calories at an elevated rate as it repairs tissues and replenishes energy stores. This is known as the "afterburn" effect or excess post-exercise oxygen consumption (EPOC). More intense and longer duration exercises generally lead to a higher EPOC effect.

4. Hormonal Influence: Exercise can impact various hormones involved in metabolism, including insulin, cortisol, and growth hormones. For example,

high-intensity exercises can improve insulin sensitivity, which can positively influence how the body processes carbohydrates.

5. Exercise and Fat Loss: Regular exercise, particularly a combination of cardiovascular and strength-training exercises, can aid in fat loss and weight management. Fat loss can contribute to improved metabolic health and a more favorable body composition.

5.2 Types of Exercises to Boost Your Metabolism

To boost metabolism effectively, a well-rounded exercise routine that includes different types of exercises is essential. Here are some types of exercises that can help enhance your metabolic rate:

1. High-Intensity Interval Training (HIIT): HIIT involves short bursts of intense exercise alternated with brief periods of rest or lower-intensity activity. It is known for its ability to increase calorie burn and elevate metabolism even after the workout is finished due to the EPOC effect. HIIT workouts can be adapted to various activities, such as running, cycling, bodyweight exercises, and more.

2. Strength Training: Resistance or strength training involves exercises that challenge your muscles, such as weightlifting or bodyweight exercises like

squats, lunges, and push-ups.
Building and maintaining
muscle mass increases BMR,
supporting overall metabolic
health.

3. Cardiovascular Exercises:
   Traditional cardiovascular
   exercises, such as running,
   cycling, swimming, and
   dancing, can help increase
   energy expenditure and
   improve cardiovascular fitness.
   These exercises contribute to a
   higher TDEE and can assist in
   weight management.

4. Circuit Training: Circuit
   training combines
   cardiovascular and strength
   exercises in a continuous
   sequence with minimal rest
   between sets. It provides both
   aerobic and anaerobic benefits,

promoting a higher calorie burn and metabolic impact.

5. Metabolic Conditioning: Metabolic conditioning workouts are designed to challenge multiple energy systems in the body, incorporating elements of strength, cardio, and plyometric exercises. These workouts can lead to increased metabolic demand and overall fitness improvements.

6. Flexibility and Mobility Exercises: While flexibility and mobility exercises may not directly increase metabolic rate, they are essential for overall fitness and well-being. Incorporating activities like yoga, Pilates, or stretching routines can support recovery

and prevent injuries, allowing you to maintain a consistent exercise routine.

7. Daily Physical Activity: Incorporating more movement into your daily life, such as taking the stairs, walking or biking instead of driving short distances, and standing rather than sitting for prolonged periods, can also contribute to increased energy expenditure and support overall metabolic health.

The most effective exercise routine is one that you enjoy and can maintain consistently. Varying your workouts and challenging your body with different exercises can help prevent plateaus and keep your metabolism engaged. Always consult with a healthcare professional or fitness expert before starting a new exercise program, especially if you have any underlying health conditions or concerns. With a balanced exercise routine and a well-rounded approach to overall health, you can effectively boost your metabolism and achieve your fitness and wellness goals.

5.3 Creating an Effective Workout Routine

Creating an effective workout routine involves careful planning and consideration of your fitness goals, fitness level, time availability, and preferences. Whether you are a beginner or experienced exerciser, a well-designed workout routine can help you achieve your desired outcomes and promote long-term fitness and overall health. Here are steps to guide you in creating an effective workout routine:

1. Set Clear Goals: Define your fitness goals. Are you looking to build strength, improve cardiovascular endurance, lose weight, increase flexibility, or a combination of these? Setting clear and specific goals will help you structure your workout routine to align with your objectives.

2. Choose the Right Exercises: Select exercises that target your specific goals and preferences. A well-rounded routine typically includes a mix of cardiovascular exercises, strength training, flexibility, and mobility exercises. Here's a breakdown:

- Cardiovascular
  Exercises: Choose
  activities that elevate
  your heart rate, such as
  running, cycling,
  swimming, dancing, or
  jumping rope. Aim for at
  least 150 minutes of
  moderate-intensity cardio
  per week or 75 minutes
  of vigorous-intensity
  cardio.

- Strength Training:
  Incorporate resistance
  exercises that target
  major muscle groups.
  You can use free
  weights, machines,
  resistance bands, or
  bodyweight exercises.
  Aim for at least two days
  of strength training per

week, with a focus on different muscle groups on separate days.

- Flexibility and Mobility Exercises: Include stretches and exercises that improve flexibility and range of motion. Yoga, Pilates, and static stretching can be beneficial for overall mobility and recovery.

3. Consider Frequency and Duration: Determine how many days per week you can commit to exercise. Aim for at least 3 to 5 days of exercise per week, with a mix of cardiovascular and strength training activities. The duration of each workout session may vary based on your fitness level and the type of

exercise you're performing. A typical workout session can range from 30 minutes to an hour.

4. Plan Your Workouts: Create a weekly workout schedule that incorporates your chosen exercises and aligns with your goals and availability. Be sure to include rest days for recovery and muscle repair. Avoid consecutive days of intense workouts to prevent overtraining and injury.

5. Gradually Progress: As you become more comfortable with your workout routine, gradually increase the intensity, duration, or frequency of your workouts. Progression is essential to challenge your body and continue making fitness gains.

6. Warm-Up and Cool-Down: Always include a warm-up before starting your main workout to prepare your body for exercise and reduce the risk of injury. Similarly, cool down after each workout to gradually lower your heart rate and stretch your muscles.

7. Listen to Your Body: Pay attention to how your body responds to the workouts. If you experience pain, fatigue, or discomfort, adjust your routine or consult with a fitness professional to ensure your exercise plan is safe and appropriate for your needs.

8. Stay Consistent: Consistency is key to achieving your fitness goals. Stick to your workout routine, even on days when

motivation is low. Having a consistent schedule will help you develop healthy exercise habits.

9. Stay Hydrated and Fuel Properly: Drink enough water before, during, and after your workouts to stay hydrated. Fuel your body with nutritious foods that provide the energy and nutrients needed to support your physical activity.

10. Be Flexible and Enjoy the Process: Be open to adjusting your routine based on your progress and preferences. Remember to have fun and enjoy the journey of improving your fitness and overall well-being.

Always consult with a healthcare professional or fitness expert before starting a new workout routine, especially if you have any health concerns or medical conditions. A certified fitness trainer or coach can also help you create a personalized workout plan tailored to your goals and fitness level.

CHAPTER 6

Lifestyle Factors Affecting Metabolism

6.1 Sleep and Its Impact on Metabolic Health

Sleep is a fundamental aspect of overall health and well-being, and it plays a significant role in metabolic health. Lack of adequate sleep or poor sleep quality can negatively affect various hormonal and physiological processes related to metabolism. Here's how sleep impacts metabolic health:

1. Hormonal Regulation: Sleep plays a crucial role in regulating hormones that affect appetite, hunger, and satiety. Poor sleep can disrupt the balance of hormones like ghrelin (which stimulates appetite) and leptin (which signals fullness), leading to increased hunger and potential overeating.

2. Insulin Sensitivity: Sleep deprivation can reduce insulin sensitivity, meaning your body may have difficulty using glucose effectively. This can contribute to higher blood sugar levels and an increased risk of insulin resistance and type 2 diabetes.

3. Cortisol and Stress Response: Lack of sleep can elevate

cortisol levels, the body's primary stress hormone. Elevated cortisol levels may contribute to metabolic disturbances, increased fat storage, and a heightened risk of metabolic syndrome.

4. Energy Balance: Inadequate sleep can lead to fatigue and reduced physical activity, which can affect overall energy balance and metabolism.

5. Thermoregulation: Sleep is essential for maintaining proper body temperature and metabolic balance.

To support metabolic health through sleep:

- Aim for 7-9 hours of quality sleep per night, as individual sleep needs may vary.

- Establish a consistent sleep schedule, going to bed and waking up at the same time each day.

- Create a relaxing bedtime routine to signal your body that it's time to wind down.

- Limit caffeine and screen time before bedtime, as they can interfere with sleep quality.

- Ensure your sleep environment is comfortable, cool, and free from distractions.

6.2 Managing Stress for a Healthy Metabolism

Chronic stress can significantly impact metabolic health. When stressed, the body releases hormones like cortisol and adrenaline, which can influence metabolism and energy balance. Prolonged stress can lead to overeating, particularly of comfort foods high in sugar and unhealthy fats, contributing to weight gain and metabolic disturbances. Here's how to manage stress for a healthy metabolism:

1. Exercise: Regular physical activity can help reduce stress and promote a positive mood. Engage in activities you enjoy, such as walking, yoga, or dancing.

2. Mindfulness and Meditation: Practice mindfulness techniques and meditation to reduce stress and promote relaxation.

3. Sleep: Prioritize quality sleep, as lack of sleep can increase stress and exacerbate its effects on metabolism.

4. Social Support: Seek support from friends, family, or a support group to help cope with stress.

5. Time Management: Organize your schedule to avoid feeling overwhelmed and stressed.

6.3 Other Lifestyle Habits to Support Your Metabolism

Beyond sleep and stress management, several other lifestyle habits can positively influence metabolism and overall health:

1. Stay Hydrated: Drink plenty of water throughout the day to support metabolism and overall well-being.

2. Eat Balanced Meals: Consume a balanced diet with a mix of macronutrients and micronutrients to support energy levels and metabolic function.

3. Avoid Crash Diets: Extreme calorie restriction or crash diets can slow down metabolism and lead to muscle loss.

4. Avoid Prolonged Sitting: Incorporate movement throughout your day, even if it's just standing up and stretching regularly.

5. Limit Alcohol and Sugary Beverages: Excessive alcohol

and sugary beverage consumption can lead to weight gain and metabolic disturbances.

6. Quit Smoking: Smoking negatively affects metabolism and overall health. If you smoke, seek support to quit.

7. Regular Physical Activity: Engage in regular exercise, including both cardiovascular activities and strength training, to support metabolic health and overall fitness.

8. Moderation in Eating: Practice portion control and avoid overeating, even if the food is healthy.

9. Be Patient and Consistent: Sustainable changes take time. Be patient with yourself and

stay consistent in adopting
healthy lifestyle habits.

Remember that everyone's metabolism is different, and lifestyle changes may affect individuals differently. Consider consulting with a healthcare professional or a registered dietitian to receive personalized advice and guidance tailored to your specific needs and goals. By prioritizing sleep, managing stress, and adopting other healthy lifestyle habits, you can support a healthy metabolism and enhance your overall well-being.

CHAPTER 7

Supercharging Your Metabolism

7.1 Intermittent Fasting and Its Effects on Metabolism

Intermittent fasting (IF) is an eating pattern that alternates between periods of eating and fasting. It has gained popularity for its potential effects on metabolism and overall health. However, it's essential to approach intermittent fasting with caution and consider individual needs and preferences. Here's how intermittent fasting may impact metabolism:

1. Insulin Sensitivity: Some studies suggest that intermittent fasting can improve insulin sensitivity, which means your body can use glucose more effectively, potentially reducing the risk of insulin resistance and type 2 diabetes.

2. Fat Burning: During fasting periods, when the body is not receiving energy from food, it may turn to stored fat for fuel. This can lead to increased fat burning and potentially contribute to weight loss.

3. Hormonal Effects: Intermittent fasting may influence hormone levels, including human growth hormone (HGH) and norepinephrine, which can support fat breakdown and metabolism.

4. Caloric Intake: IF can lead to reduced caloric intake, especially if eating periods are shorter or less frequent. A caloric deficit can result in weight loss, which may improve metabolic health.

It's important to note that intermittent fasting is not suitable for everyone. It may not be recommended for individuals with certain medical conditions, pregnant or breastfeeding women, individuals with a history of disordered eating, or those who struggle with low blood sugar levels. If you are considering intermittent fasting, consult with a healthcare professional or registered dietitian to ensure it's safe and appropriate for your individual needs.

7.2 Metabolism-Enhancing Supplements

While some supplements claim to boost metabolism, it's essential to approach such claims with skepticism. The effectiveness and safety of metabolism-enhancing supplements vary, and not all products deliver the promised results. Here are some commonly marketed metabolism-boosting supplements and their potential impact:

1. Caffeine: Caffeine is a central nervous system stimulant found in coffee, tea, energy drinks, and some supplements. It can temporarily increase metabolic rate and fat oxidation. However, the effects may diminish with regular use, and excessive caffeine intake can lead to adverse side effects.

2. Green Tea Extract: Green tea contains compounds like catechins and caffeine that may enhance thermogenesis (calorie burning). Green tea extract supplements are marketed for their potential metabolism-boosting effects.

3. Capsaicin (from chili peppers): Some studies suggest that capsaicin may increase metabolic rate and promote fat oxidation. It is commonly found in weight loss supplements.

4. L-Carnitine: L-Carnitine is an amino acid involved in fat metabolism and energy production. Some believe that supplementing with L-Carnitine can increase fat burning, but research results are mixed.

5. Conjugated Linoleic Acid (CLA): CLA is a type of fatty acid found in meat and dairy products. It is often promoted as a fat-burning supplement, but research on its effectiveness is inconclusive.

It's important to approach supplements with caution and consult with a healthcare professional before adding them to your regimen. Many metabolism-enhancing supplements lack sufficient scientific evidence to support their effectiveness or safety. Focus on a well-rounded diet, regular exercise, and lifestyle habits that promote overall health and metabolic function.

7.3 Other Strategies for Revving Up Your Metabolism

In addition to intermittent fasting and supplements, several other strategies can potentially enhance your metabolism and overall well-being:

1. Stay Active: Regular physical activity, including both cardiovascular exercises and strength training, can help boost metabolism and maintain muscle mass.

2. Stay Hydrated: Drinking enough water can support metabolic function and help prevent dehydration.

3. Eat Protein-Rich Foods: Protein has a higher thermic effect, meaning it requires more

energy to digest, helping to slightly increase metabolism.

4. Eat Smaller, Frequent Meals: Some people find that eating smaller, more frequent meals can help maintain energy levels and control appetite.

5. Incorporate Spicy Foods: Capsaicin in spicy foods may temporarily boost metabolism and increase fat burning.

6. Optimize Thyroid Health: Ensure proper thyroid function, as the thyroid hormone plays a crucial role in metabolism.

7. Reduce Sedentary Time: Avoid prolonged sitting and incorporate movement throughout your day.

8. Get Enough Vitamin D: Vitamin D deficiency may be linked to slower metabolism; consider getting enough sunlight or taking supplements if needed.

9. Avoid Crash Diets: Extreme diets or very low-calorie intake can slow down metabolism.

10. Manage Stress: Chronic stress can impact metabolism, so practice stress-reduction techniques.

It's essential to remember that individual responses to these strategies may vary. Sustainable lifestyle changes, such as maintaining a balanced diet, staying physically active, getting enough sleep, and managing stress, are essential for supporting a healthy metabolism and overall well-being. Focus on long-term habits that promote health rather than quick fixes or drastic measures. Consult with a healthcare professional or registered dietitian for personalized advice and guidance based on your individual needs and goals.

CHAPTER 8

Overcoming Metabolism Challenges

8.1 Plateaus and How to Break Through Them

Experiencing plateaus in weight loss or progress during your fitness journey is common, and it can be frustrating. Plateaus occur when your body adapts to your current routine, leading to a slowdown in results. Overcoming metabolism challenges and breaking through plateaus require a strategic approach. Here are some tips to help you overcome plateaus:

1. Reevaluate Your Caloric
   Intake: As you lose weight,
   your calorie needs may
   decrease. Recalculate your
   daily calorie needs and adjust
   your intake accordingly to
   ensure you maintain a calorie
   deficit for weight loss.

2. Change Your Workout
   Routine: Modify your exercise
   program to challenge your body
   differently. Add variety to your
   workouts, incorporate new
   exercises, increase intensity, or
   try a different form of exercise
   to keep your body guessing.

3. Increase Strength Training:
   Increasing muscle mass
   through strength training can
   boost your metabolism, as
   muscles require more energy
   for maintenance. Consider

adding more strength training
sessions or increasing the
intensity of your current
workouts.

4. Incorporate High-Intensity
   Interval Training (HIIT): HIIT
   workouts can be effective for
   breaking through plateaus by
   increasing calorie burn and
   elevating metabolism both
   during and after exercise.

5. Watch Your Portions: Be
   mindful of portion sizes and
   avoid mindless eating. Even
   healthy foods can contribute to
   weight gain if consumed in
   excess.

6. Manage Stress: Chronic stress
   can impact hormones and
   metabolism. Implement stress-
   reduction techniques like

mindfulness, meditation, or hobbies you enjoy.

7. Prioritize Sleep: Ensure you're getting enough quality sleep, as sleep deprivation can affect hormones and hinder weight loss progress.

8. Monitor Your Progress: Keep track of your food intake, exercise routine, and progress. Monitoring your efforts can help you identify areas for improvement and stay motivated.

9. Stay Hydrated: Drinking enough water can support your metabolism and help you feel full, potentially reducing overeating.

10. Be Patient and Persistent: Plateaus are a natural part of

the process. Stay committed to your goals, and remember that sustainable progress takes time and consistency.

8.2 Dealing with Metabolism Changes as You Age

Metabolism naturally changes as we age, which can influence body composition and weight management. Several factors contribute to these changes:

1. Muscle Loss: With age, there is a gradual loss of muscle mass, which can lead to a decrease in basal metabolic rate (BMR). To combat muscle loss, prioritize strength training exercises to maintain and build muscle.

2. Hormonal Changes: Hormonal fluctuations, particularly in menopause for women and andropause for men, can impact metabolism and weight distribution. Regular exercise and a balanced diet can help mitigate the effects of hormonal changes.

3. Lifestyle and Activity Levels: As people age, their activity levels may decrease, leading to reduced daily energy expenditure. Engaging in regular physical activity can help counteract this decline in metabolism.

4. Nutrient Needs: Older adults may require fewer calories due to changes in activity levels and body composition. Ensure you

are meeting your nutrient needs with a nutrient-dense diet.

Tips for managing metabolism changes as you age:

1. Stay Active: Regular exercise, including cardiovascular and strength training, can help maintain muscle mass and support metabolic health.

2. Prioritize Protein: Adequate protein intake is essential for maintaining muscle mass and supporting metabolic function.

3. Focus on Nutrient-Dense Foods: Choose whole, nutrient-dense foods to ensure you're getting the necessary nutrients without excess calories.

4. Monitor Caloric Intake: Adjust your caloric intake to match

your activity level and changing metabolic needs.

5. Stay Hydrated: Drinking enough water is essential for overall health and can support metabolic function.

6. Get Adequate Sleep: Quality sleep is vital for hormonal regulation and overall well-being.

7. Manage Stress: Chronic stress can impact metabolism and overall health, so practice stress management techniques.

Aging is a natural process, and while metabolism may change, making healthy lifestyle choices can help maintain overall well-being and manage any age-related metabolic challenges. If you have specific concerns about your metabolism or

weight management, consult with a
healthcare professional or a registered
dietitian for personalized guidance
and support.

CHAPTER 9

Designing Your Personalized Metabolism Plan

9.1 Setting Realistic Goals

Designing a personalized metabolism plan begins with setting realistic and achievable goals. Whether your focus is weight loss, improving fitness, or enhancing overall metabolic health, setting specific and attainable goals is crucial for success. Here's how to set realistic goals:

1. Be Specific: Define your goals clearly. For example, instead of

saying "I want to lose weight," specify how much weight you aim to lose and in what timeframe.

2. Make It Measurable: Set quantifiable metrics to track your progress. This could be the number of pounds lost, the number of inches reduced, or improvements in strength and endurance.

3. Set Achievable Targets: Ensure your goals are realistic and attainable. Consider your current fitness level, lifestyle, and time commitments when setting your targets.

4. Be Time-Bound: Establish a timeframe for achieving your goals. Having a deadline can

provide motivation and help you stay focused.

5. Break Down Larger Goals: If you have significant long-term goals, break them down into smaller, manageable milestones. Celebrate your achievements along the way to maintain motivation.

6. Consider Non-Scale Goals: Don't solely focus on the scale. Set non-scale goals, such as increasing the number of push-ups you can do or improving your running pace.

9.2 Creating a Sustainable and Enjoyable Plan

A successful metabolism plan should be sustainable and enjoyable, promoting long-term adherence and positive lifestyle changes. Here's how to create a plan that fits your needs:

1. Identify Activities You Enjoy: Choose exercises and physical activities you genuinely enjoy, whether it's dancing, hiking, swimming, or cycling. Enjoyable activities are more likely to become habits.

2. Find Balance in Nutrition: Create a balanced and varied diet that includes foods you love while also meeting your nutritional needs. Avoid

extreme diets that are difficult to maintain.

3. Set Realistic Exercise Frequency: Plan an exercise routine that aligns with your schedule and energy levels. Consistency is more important than extreme workout schedules.

4. Incorporate Rest Days: Allow ample time for rest and recovery to prevent burnout and injury. Rest is essential for muscle repair and overall well-being.

5. Join Supportive Communities: Consider joining fitness classes, online groups, or partnering with a workout buddy. Surrounding yourself with

supportive individuals can keep you motivated and accountable.

6. Be Flexible: Life is unpredictable, and there will be days when your plan may need to adapt. Be flexible and willing to adjust your schedule and goals as needed.

9.3 Tracking Your Progress and Making Adjustments

Tracking your progress is essential for assessing your metabolism plan's effectiveness and making necessary adjustments. Here's how to track your progress and make changes:

1. Keep a Journal: Maintain a journal to record your

workouts, meals, energy levels, and emotions. This can help you identify patterns and make informed decisions.

2. Track Measurements: Regularly measure your weight, body measurements, and fitness performance to monitor changes and celebrate your successes.

3. Monitor Energy Levels: Pay attention to how you feel throughout the day. Adequate nutrition and rest should support your energy levels and overall well-being.

4. Assess Your Goals: Periodically evaluate your progress toward your goals. Celebrate achievements and

reassess if needed to set new targets or adjust your plan.

5. Consult Professionals: If you encounter challenges or have specific health concerns, consider seeking guidance from a healthcare professional, registered dietitian, or certified fitness trainer.

6. Stay Positive and Patient: Progress may not always be linear, and you might face setbacks. Stay positive, be patient with yourself, and focus on the journey rather than perfection.

A personalized metabolism plan is unique to you. What works for someone else may not work for you, and that's okay. Listen to your body, stay committed to your goals, and

make adjustments as needed to create
a plan that supports your health and
well-being for the long term.

www.ingramcontent.com/pod-product-compliance
Lightning Source LLC
Chambersburg PA
CBHW070853260726

48661CB00004B/1389